What ha
when y
LISTE

Published by Evans Brothers Limited
2A Portman Mansions
Chiltern Street
London W1M 1LE

First published in Great Britain in 1985 by
Hamish Hamilton Children's Books

© Joy Richardson (text) 1985

© Colin and Moira Maclean (illustrations) 1985

All Rights Reserved. No part of this publication may be reproduced, stored in a retrieval system or transmitted in any form or by any means, electronic, mechanical, photocopying or otherwise, without prior permission of Evans Brothers Limited.

Reprinted 1986
New edition published 1992

The author and publishers would like to thank Dr R. H. James MB, BS, FFARCS for his help and advice with the preparation of this book.

Typeset by Katerprint Co. Ltd, Oxford
Printed in Hong Kong

ISBN 0 237 60206 7

What happens when you LISTEN?

Joy Richardson

Illustrated by
Colin and Moira Maclean

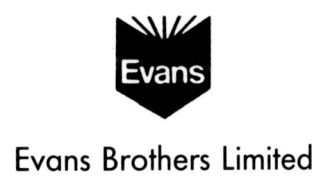

Evans Brothers Limited

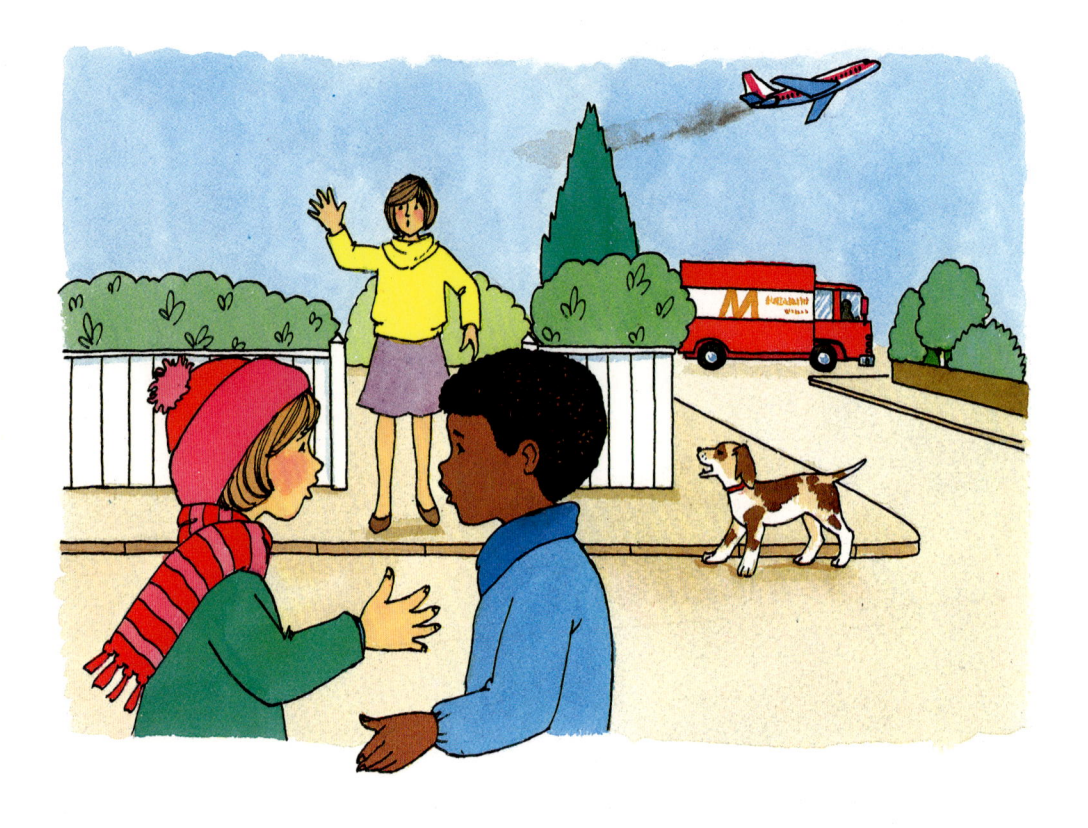

Your ears never close.
They collect sounds all day long
and pass them on to your brain.

Your brain thinks about the sounds.
It tells you which ones
to listen to.

Sounds travel through the air
to get to your ears.
Sounds make the air vibrate
(shake up and down very fast).

Hook an elastic band over a
door handle and stretch it out.
Pluck the elastic band and watch it vibrate
while it makes a sound.

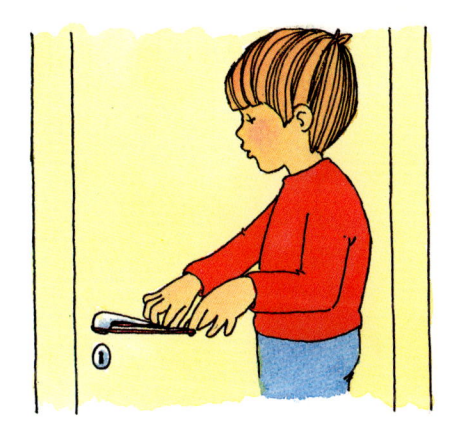

When the elastic band vibrates
it sets off vibrations in the air.
The vibrations in the air carry
the sound to your ears.

Fill a large bowl with water.
Let drops of water fall from a teaspoon
into the middle of the bowl.
Watch the ripples spreading out.

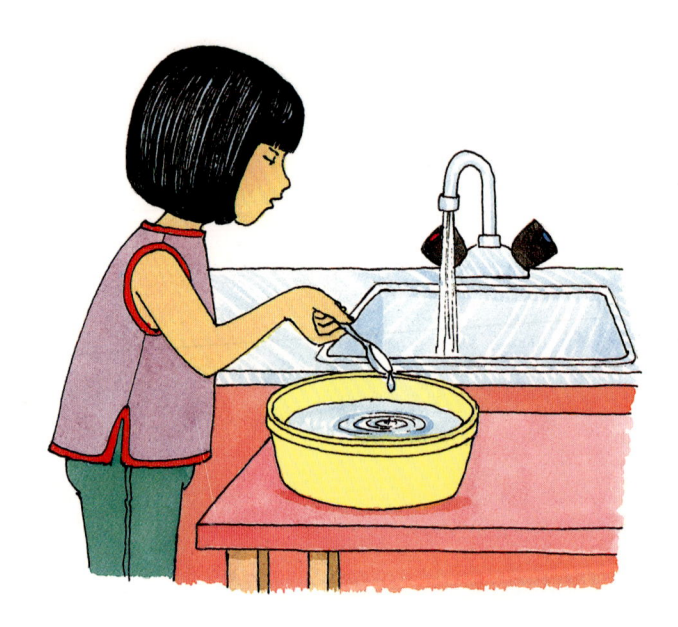

Sounds make ripples in the air.
They are called sound waves.
They spread out in all directions.
So when you make a noise,
people all round you can hear it.

Sound waves can travel round corners.
They can travel through windows and walls.
As they travel they get weaker.
In the end they fade away.

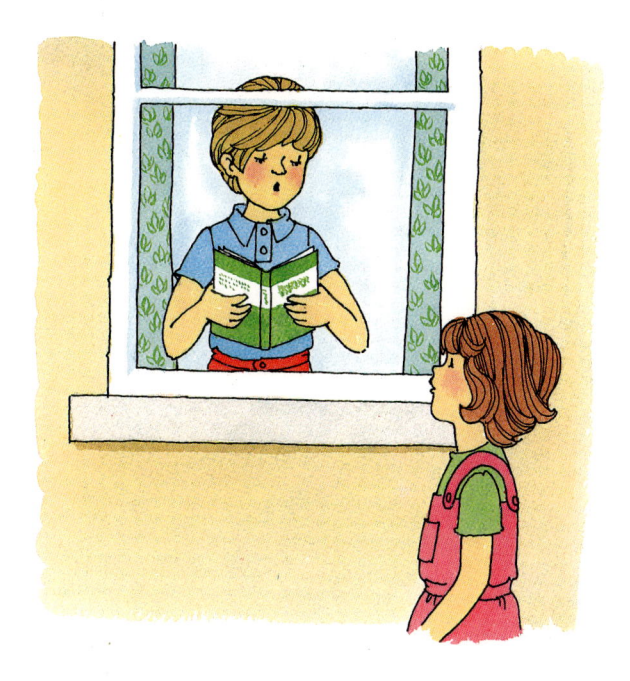

Listen to a friend saying a nursery rhyme.
Now find a place where you can
only hear it faintly.
Find a place where you
cannot hear it at all.

Animals like dogs and rabbits
can prick their ears up
to help catch the sound waves.
Try wiggling your ears.
You cannot move your ears much
but they are a good shape
for collecting sounds.

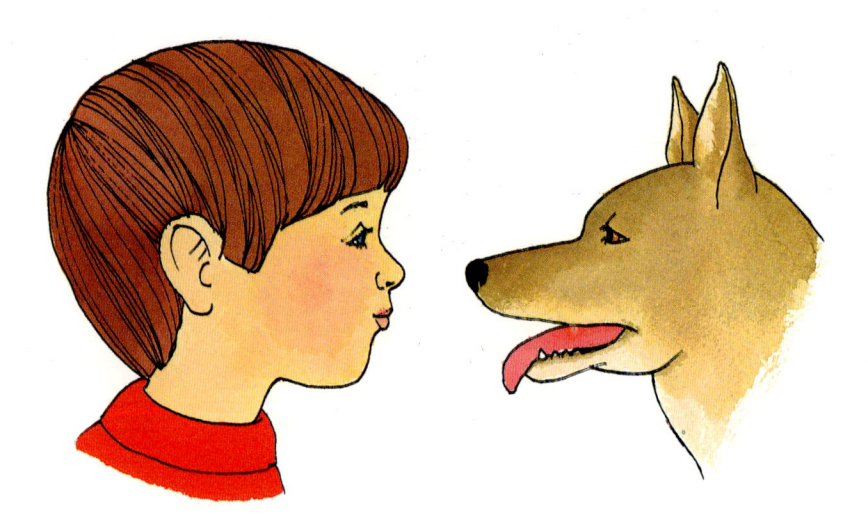

Cut half a circle out of
a piece of thin card.
Stick the ends of the straight edge
together to make a funnel.
Stick the pointed end round
the end of a toilet roll tube.
Use your funnel
to listen to nearby sounds.

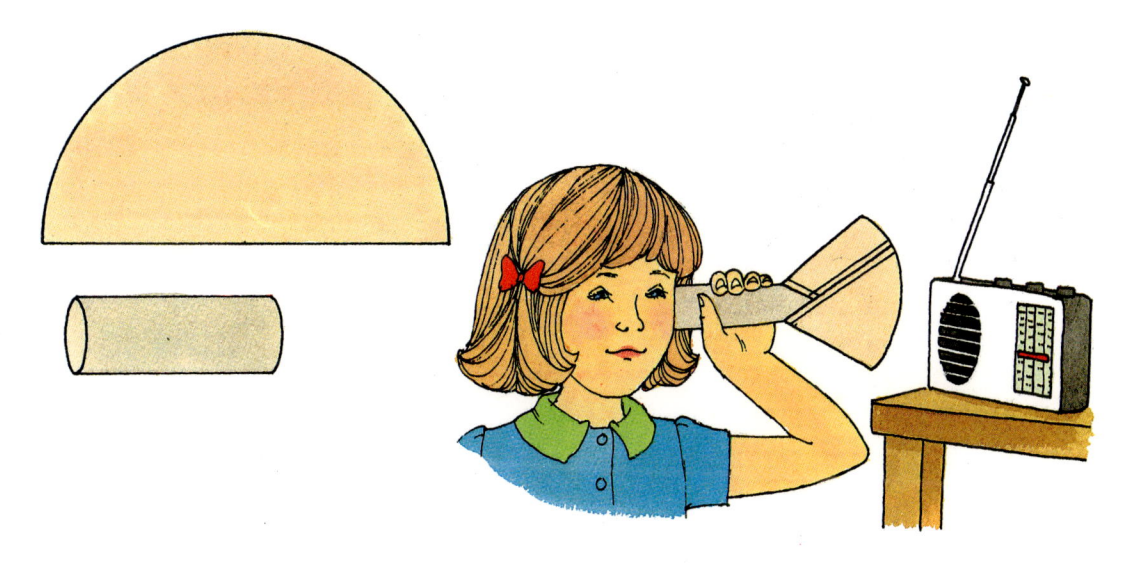

Your ear is like a funnel.
There is a wide opening
on the side of your head
and a narrow tube inside.

Sound waves travel along a
narrow tube inside your ear.

Hold a tube of card to your ear.
Ask a friend to talk down the tube.
Now listen to your friend
without the tube.

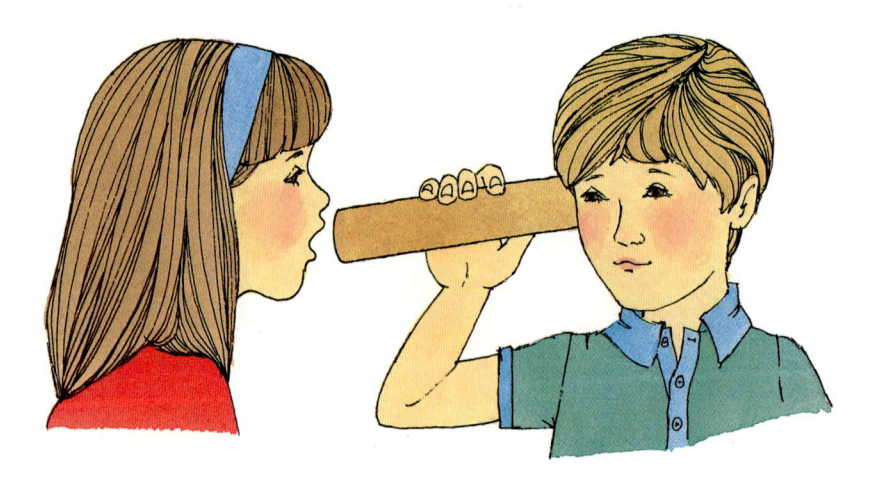

The sound is louder down the tube
because the sound waves cannot spread out.

ear —

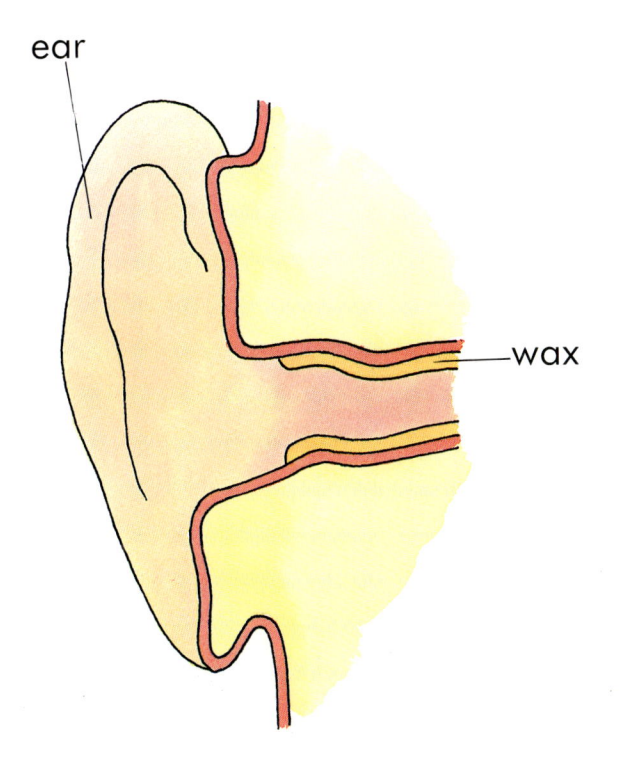

wax —

Put your little finger
gently into your ear.
Feel the opening of the tube.
Is it sticky?

The walls of the tube
make a sticky yellow wax.
The wax traps dust.

8

Sound waves travel about
two centimetres along the tube.
Then they come to your eardrum.
Your eardrum is a thin skin
across the end of the tube.

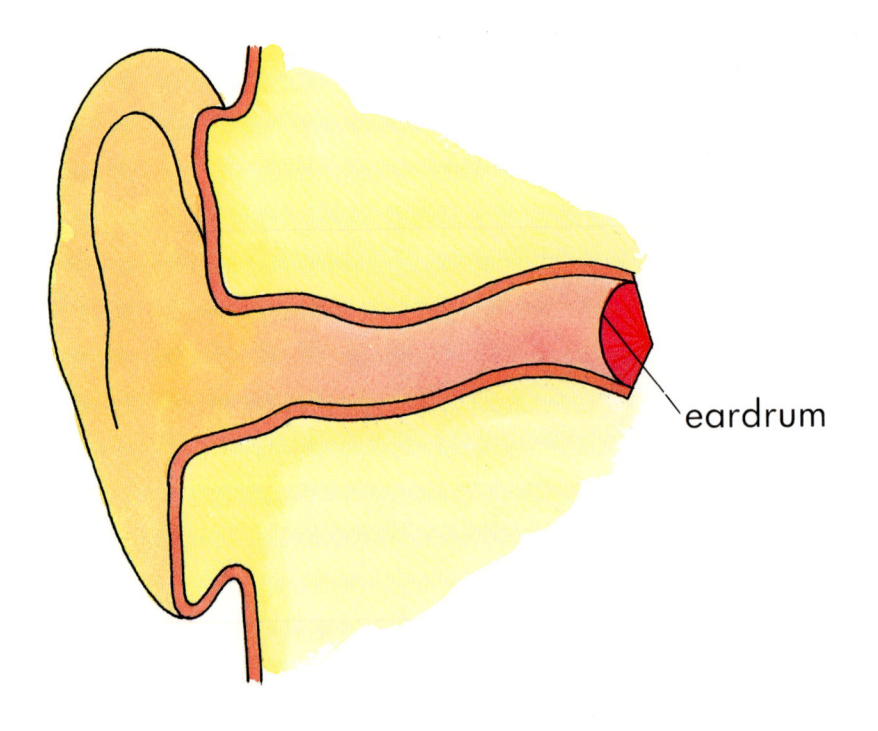

eardrum

Fix a piece of paper over
the end of a toilet roll tube
with an elastic band.
Hold one finger across the paper
so that it touches it lightly.
Talk or sing into the
open end of the tube.
What does your finger feel?

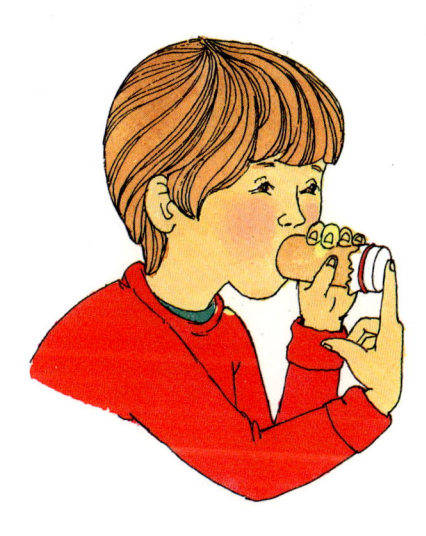

Sound waves travel through
the air in the tube.
They make the paper vibrate.
The vibrations pass through the paper
and into your finger.

bone

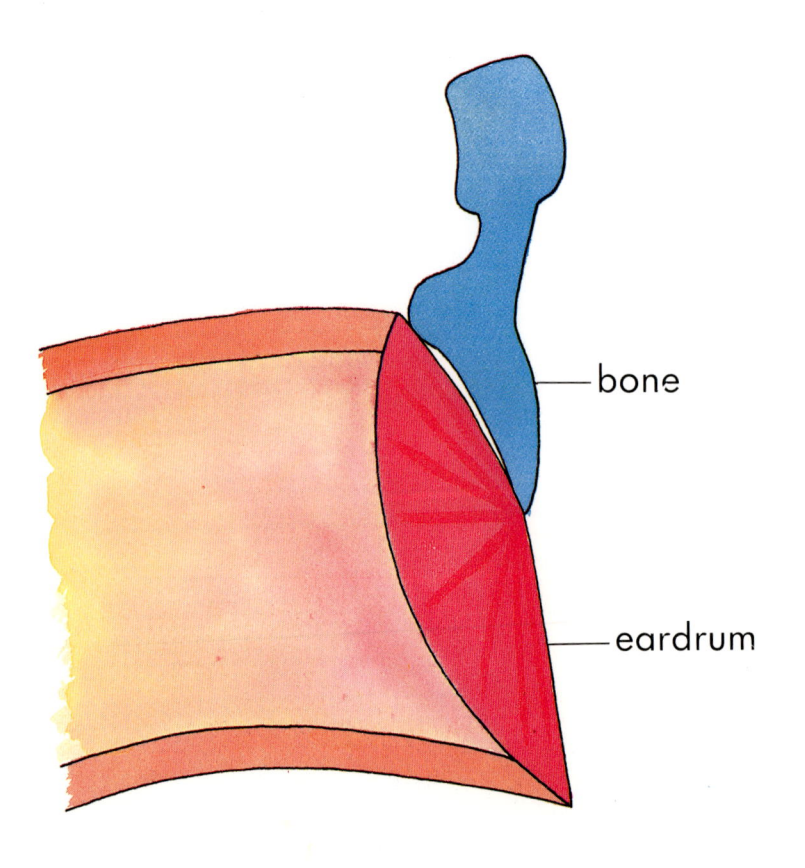

eardrum

Sound waves make your eardrum vibrate.
On the other side of your eardrum
there are three tiny bones.
Your eardrum touches the
end of the first bone
and makes it vibrate too.

The first bone touches
the second bone
and makes it vibrate.
The second bone touches
the third bone
and makes it vibrate.

The vibrations get stronger
as they travel through the bones.

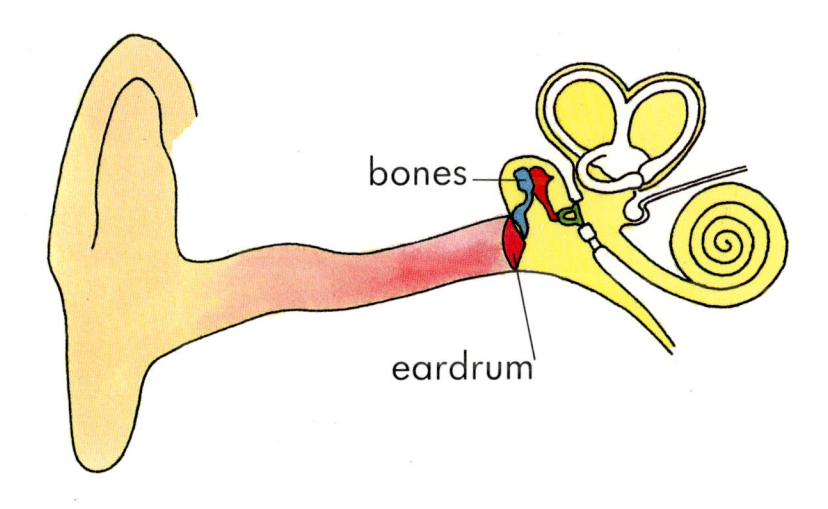

bones

eardrum

The vibrations pass into a tube filled with liquid.
The tube curls round into a spiral like a snail's shell.

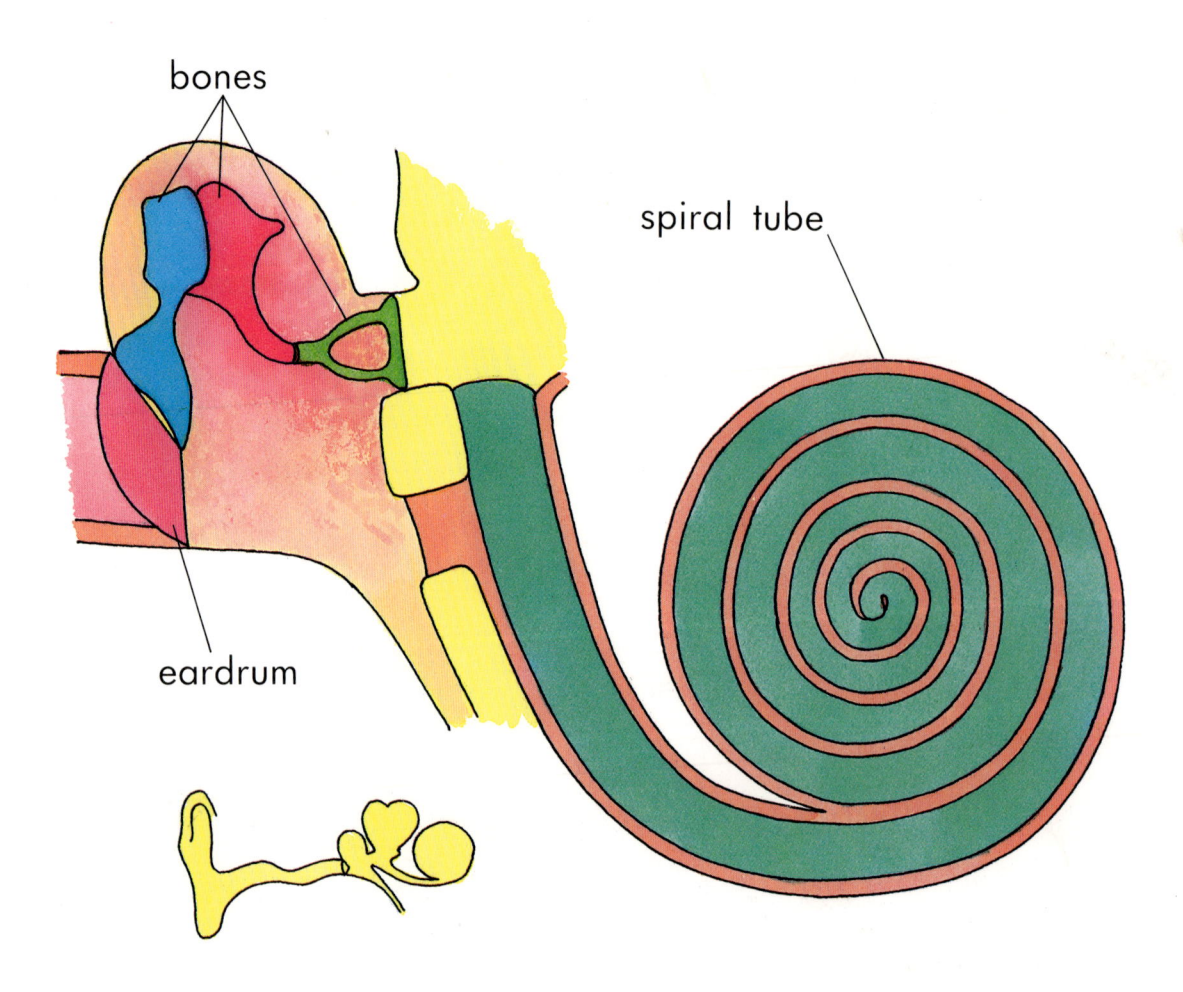

bones

spiral tube

eardrum

13

hairs inside
the spiral tube

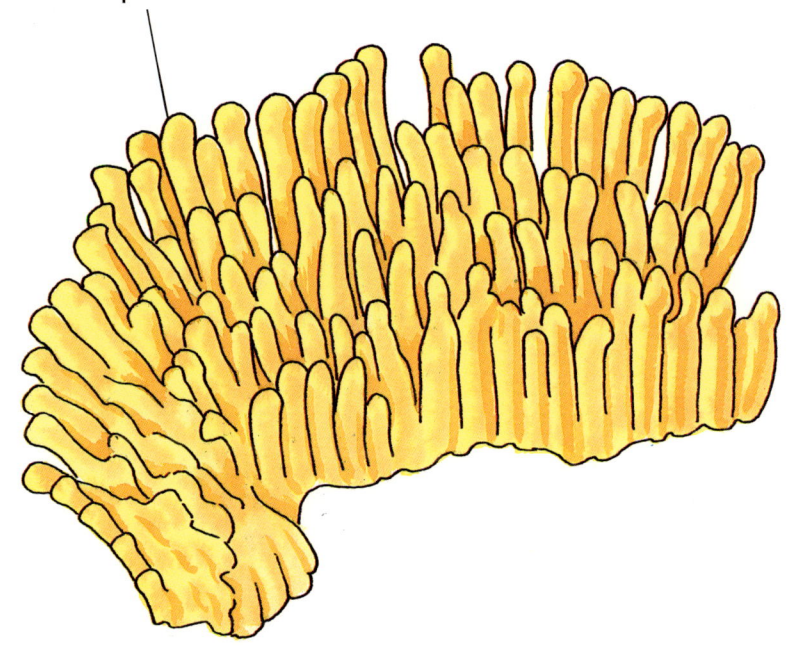

The spiral tube is lined with hairs.
When the liquid vibrates
it makes the hairs move.

High sounds make the hairs move
near the beginning of the spiral.
Low sounds make the hairs move
near the end of the spiral.

Thin threads called nerves
run from the ends of the hairs.
When a hair moves,
the nerve picks up a message
about the sound.

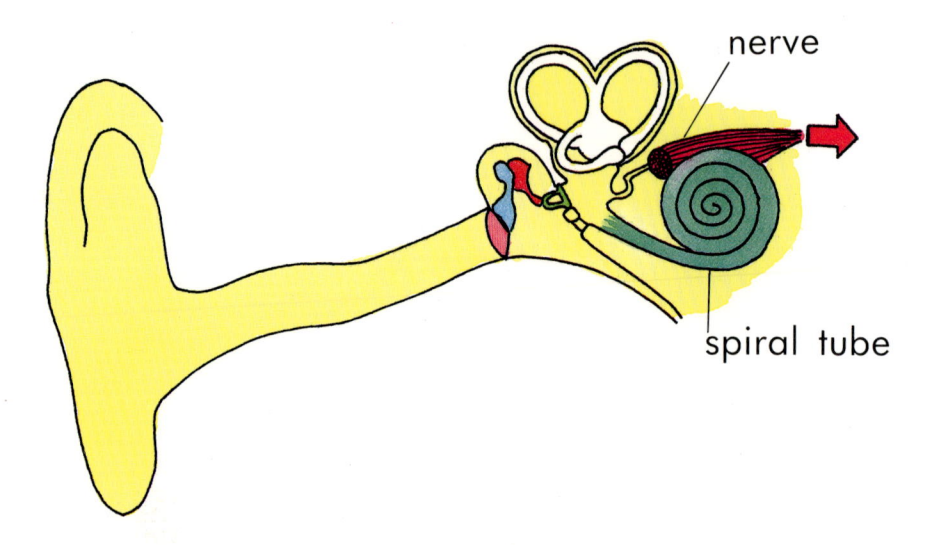

nerve

spiral tube

The nerves join up
into a big nerve.
It carries all the messages
to your brain.
Your brain works out
what the sound is like.

Your brain can work out
where a sound is coming from.

Sit on the floor
with your eyes closed.
Ask some friends to stand round you
and say your name one at a time.
Point to where you think
the sound is coming from.

How many times were you right?

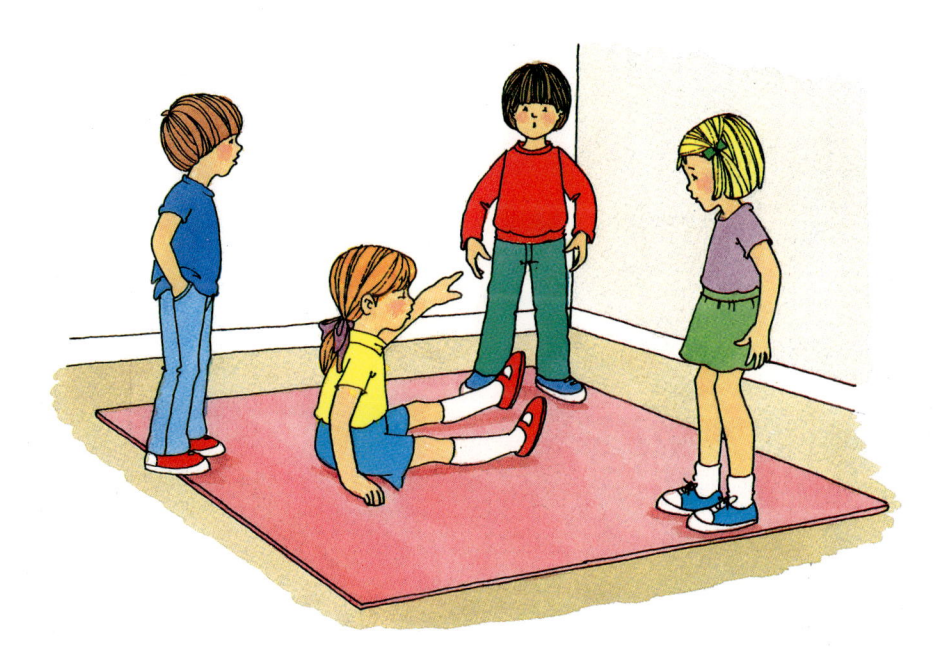

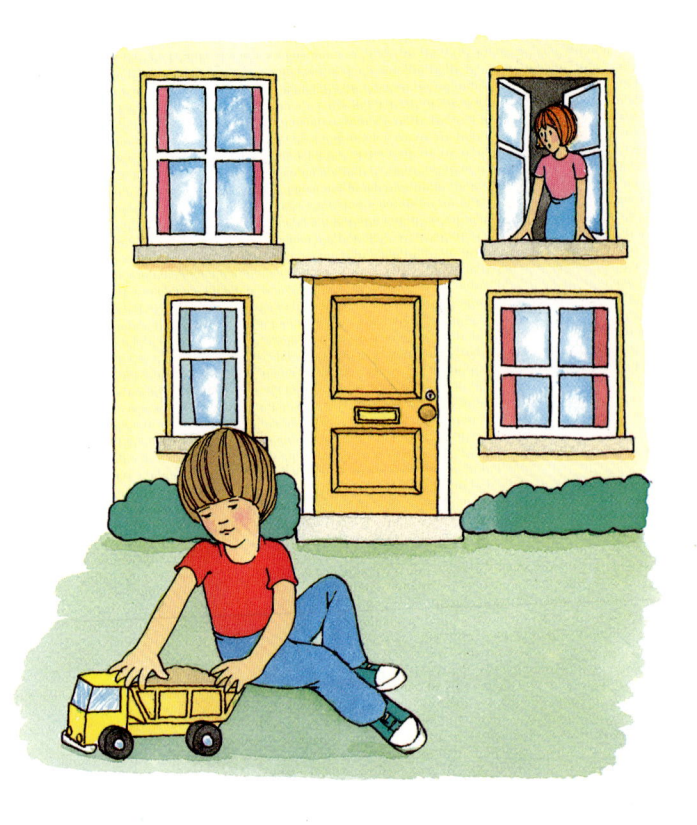

Your brain gets messages
from both your ears.
The ear which is closest to the sound
hears it first.
This helps your brain to work out
where the sound is coming from.

You listen with your ears,
but they also help you
to keep your balance.

Near the spiral tube there are
some little bags and rings
filled with liquid.
When you move your head
this liquid moves around.

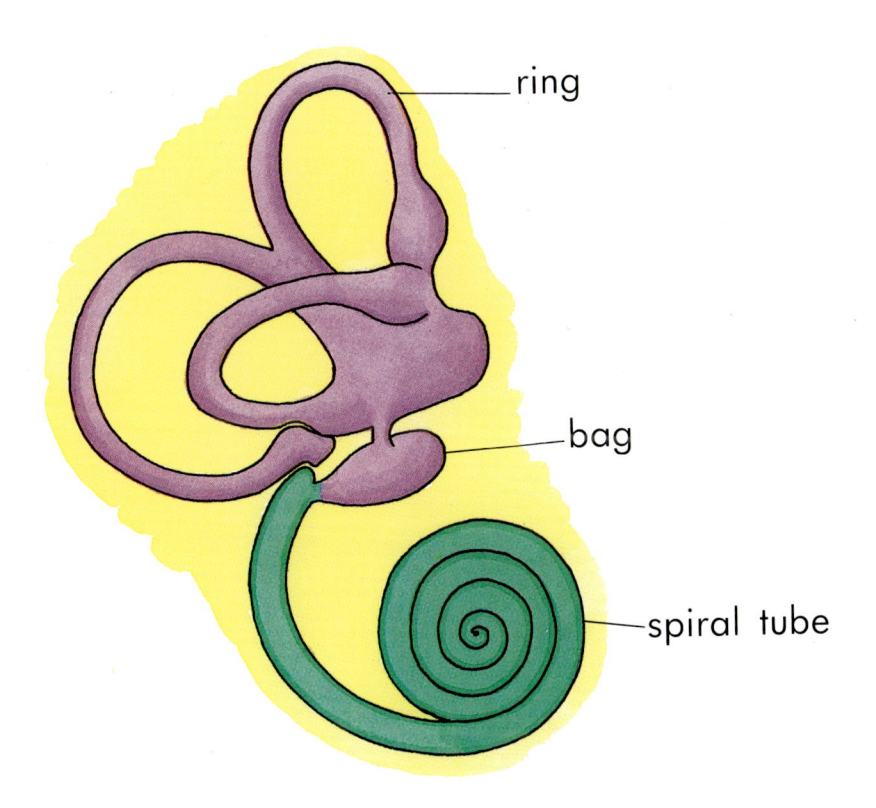

ring

bag

spiral tube

Put a spoonful of rice
into a jam jar full of water.
Screw the lid on.
Tip the jar up and down
and sideways.
What happens to the rice?

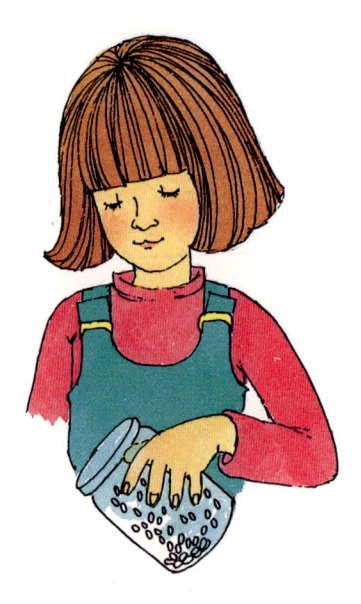

There are tiny crystals
in the liquid in the balance bags.
When you move your head
they sink to the lowest place,
like the rice in the jam jar.

When the crystals land, they
press on the ends of nerves.
The nerves tell your brain
how your head is moving.

If you twist round very fast
the balance bags get confused.
It is difficult to keep your balance.

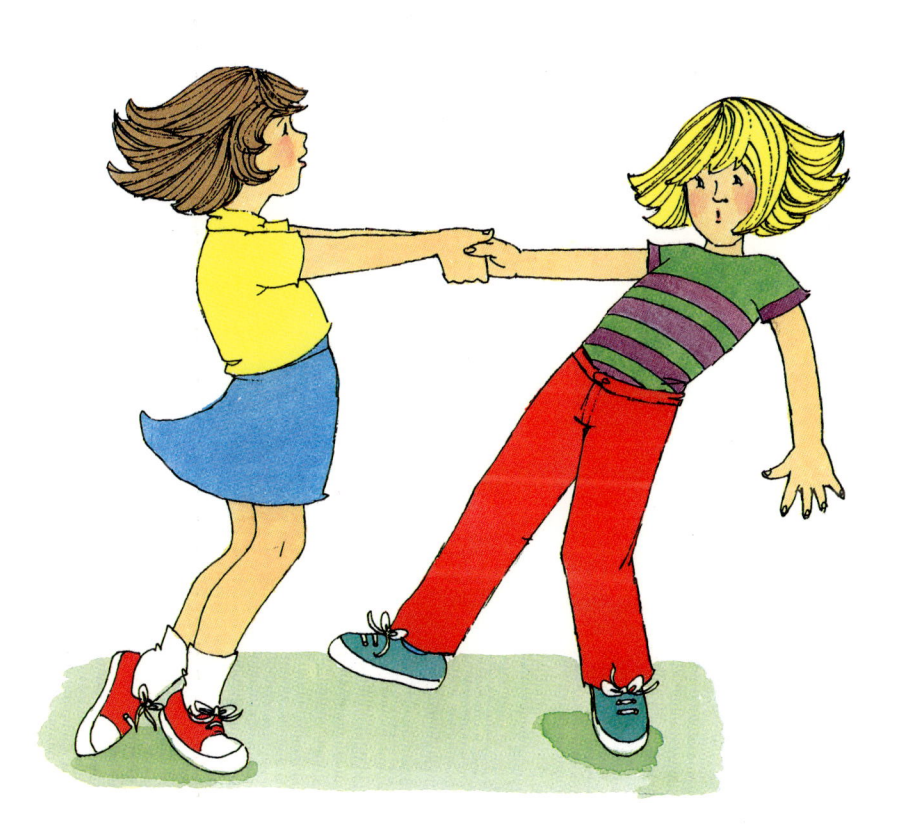

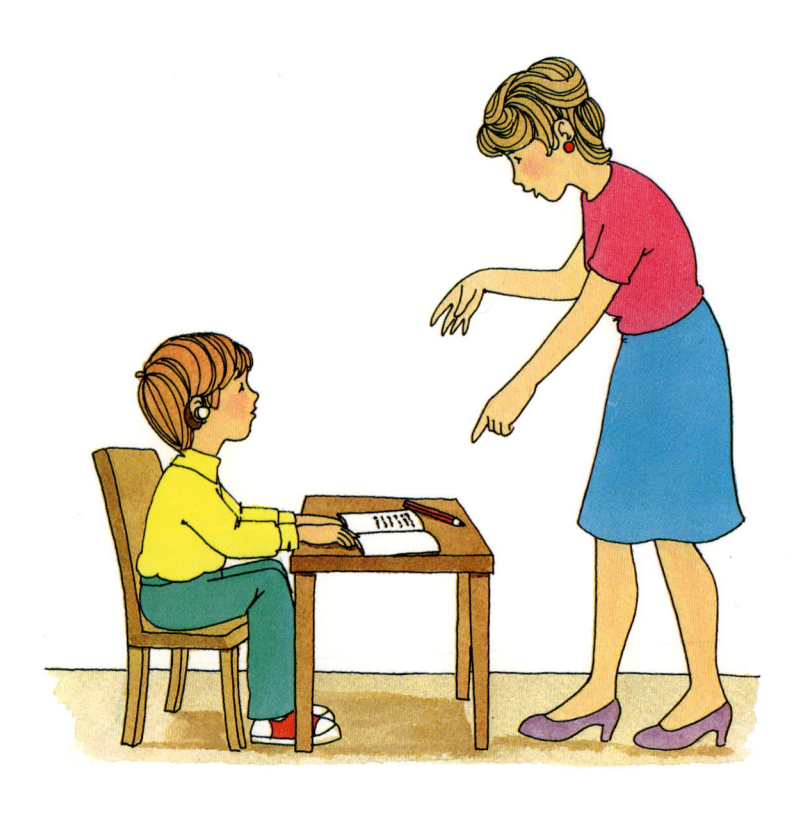

Deaf people cannot hear properly.
The nerves in their ears
do not pick up clear messages.

They may wear hearing aids
to make the sounds stronger
inside their ears.

There is a narrow tube
from your throat to your ear.
Air needs to get through the tube
to let your eardrum vibrate.

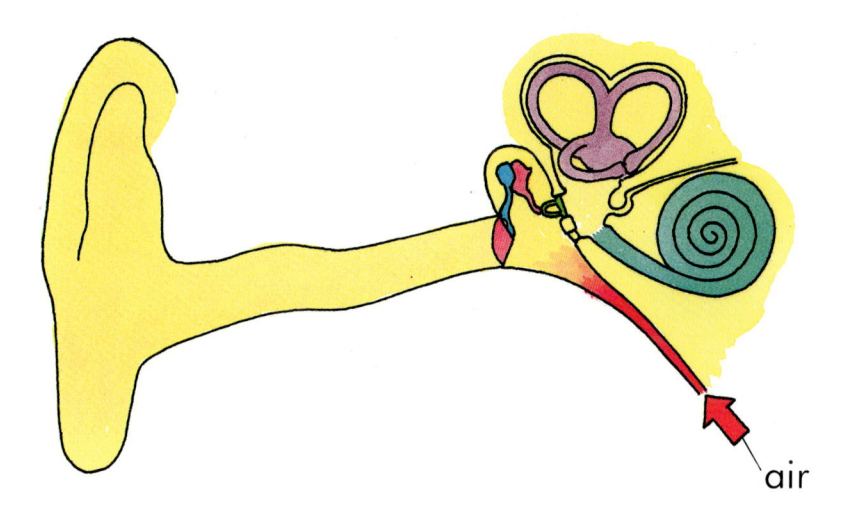

air

If you have a cold, you may not
be able to hear very well.
This is because the tube is blocked.

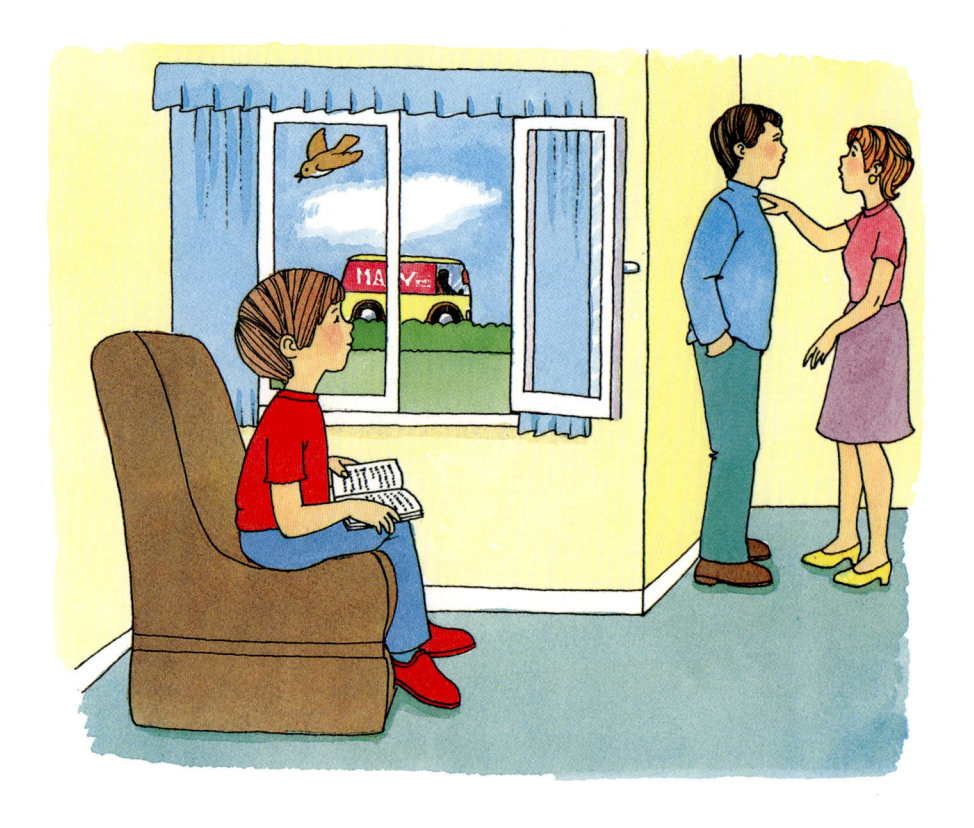

Your ears collect lots of sounds.
You are too busy
to listen to all of them.

Put this book down and listen hard.
How many sounds can you hear now?

INDEX

balance	19–21
brain	2, 16, 17, 18
deafness	22
ear, design of	7–8
eardrum	10, 12, 23
nerves	16, 21
sound waves	4, 5, 6, 8, 10, 11, 12
vibrations	3, 11, 12, 13, 14, 15
wax	9